DIY Makeup and Pro

The All Natural, Chemical Free Cosmetics Book

By: Julia Broderick

Table of Contents

Introduction
Chapter 1: The Cosmetic Industry
Chapter 2: Toxic Ingredients in Your Makeup
Chapter 3: Guidelines for Oils and Skin Types
Chapter 4: Homemade Foundation
Chapter 5: Homemade Blush
Chapter 6: DIY Bronzer
Chapter 7: DIY Eyeliner
Chapter 8: DIY Mascara
Chapter 9: DIY Eye Shadow
Chapter 10: DIY Primer
Chapter 11: Homemade Cleansers and Moisturizers
Chapter 12: DIY Toners
Chapter 13: DIY Face Masks
Chapter 14: Shampoo/Conditioner & Hair Treatments
Chapter 15: Lip and Body Scrubs
Chapter 16: Homemade Hairspray
Chapter 17: DIY Lipstick and Lip Gloss
Conclusion

For a FREE copy of my book;

Face Mask Recipes *60 Homemade Face Mask Recipes For Beautiful, Radiant Skin*

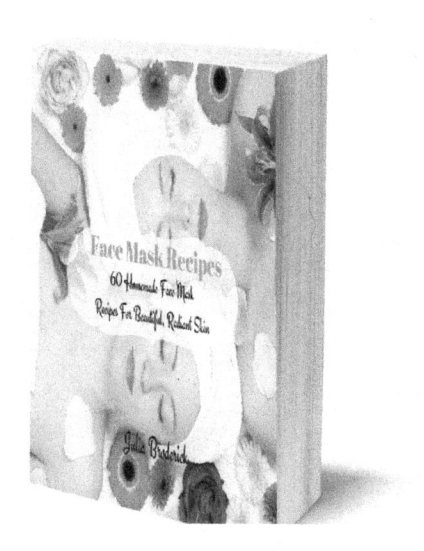

Type the link below into your internet browser:

http://eepurl.com/bWMRZb

Julia Broderick Social Media;

Website/blog:

http://www.beautifulhealthymom.com/

Youtube Channel:

https://www.youtube.com/user/beautifulhealthymom1

Facebook Page;

https://www.facebook.com/BeautifulHealthyMom/

Twitter:

https://twitter.com/Beautyhealthmom

For more books;

http://www.beautifulhealthymom.com/our-products/

© **Copyright 2015 by Julia Broderick - All rights reserved.**

It is illegal to reproduce, transmit or duplicate any part of this document through any printing or electronic means. Recording or duplication of this publication is strictly prohibited by law as well as any storage of this document, unless there is written consent on the part of the intellectual property rights holder. All rights reserved.

The author and/or intellectual property rights holder is not to be held liable for any of the information used or misused in this book. Anyone who uses or misuses the information contained within this e-book does so at their own risk. If any health issues or other problems result the author and/or intellectual property rights holder is not to be held liable for the said problem. If the information is used by anyone reading this book, the person should understand it is entirely at his/her own discretion and thereby relieving the author of any responsibility.

Introduction

You can turn your wrinkles into something unseen. It is possible to protect your skin with just a few ingredients. You can also change the shape of your face with the right touch of makeup. Makeup is an amazing creation, but it has turned into one where manufacturers use synthetic ingredients that often have toxic roots. Fortunately, you can stop harming your skin by using the information in this eBook.

You now have several recipes at your fingertips and many that you can experiment with to fit your skin and personal needs. All it takes is a little enthusiasm, a few hours in your kitchen, and good music. Perhaps you will want to invite a few friends over to make a party out of your DIY Makeup fiesta.

All of the recipes in this book have been chosen properly, based on their properties and qualities, to ensure that you are not damaging your skin or health with improper ingredients. The recipes in this book were crafted with simple steps. As you read, you will discover that some recipes only need a couple of base ingredients and essential oils or plant additives to make beautiful makeup, lotions, cosmetics, and much more.

Others might require you to shop around for the ingredients such as essential oils, butters, and beeswax. When purchased organically, these ingredients are toxic free, safe to use, and usually simple to find.

The truth is, you don't even have to step out of your kitchen for most of the makeup and other beauty products discussed in the chapters of this book. Many can be crafted from the flowers and plants that you already grow around your home and things like ground cinnamon, cornstarch, or cocoa powder.

There are 20 chapters in this eBook, each delving into various makeup and cosmetic applications. You will also find homemade beauty products such as: DIY creams, scrubs, foundations, blushes, eye shadows, eye liners, mascaras, lipsticks and much more. If kept in the fridge, most of these DIY makeup products will last around a week or two. The best advice I can give you is to be your own judge; if it no longer looks or feels fresh, throw it away.

It is important that you have a coffee grinder on hand when creating these products. It is crucial to grind the mentioned powders together in a coffee grinder in order to achieve the perfect texture. I also recommend that you do a patch test on your face and the sensitive parts of your skin to ensure that you are not allergic or intolerant to any of the ingredients that are mentioned in this book. Discover how you can make fun DIY makeup recipes that contain only natural, 100% safe ingredients to ensure your skin and hair remain beautiful throughout your lifetime.

Chapter 1: The Cosmetic Industry

The cosmetic industry is controlled by only a few multi-national corporations around the globe. The biggest section of cosmetic sales is in skincare, accounting for 33.8% of the products sold on the global market as of 2012.

Despite or perhaps because of the sheer size of the industry, it is not as regulated as you might think. Each country has their own specific regulations, including the USA under the Food and Drug Administration. The FDA states that any products intended to be sprinkled, poured, rubbed, sprayed on or otherwise applied to the body for beautifying, cleansing, altering appearance, or prompting attractiveness are considered cosmetics. This includes perms, facial makeup, eye makeup, lipsticks, perfumes, skin moisturizers, hair colors, deodorants, and shampoos. It does not include soap.

The act also states that if the product is meant to treat or prevent disease, then it is considered a drug or medical device, which has other laws and regulations. However, personal care products, such as those named in the previous paragraph, are not meant to be preventative or to treat any disease. They are also not considered dietary supplements in most cases.

The cosmetic industry is different with regards to FDA legal authority. By law, cosmetic ingredients and products are not subject to pre-market approval unless they contain color additives. This means a cosmetic product can enter the sales market without being approved or tested by the FDA. It is required to have a label, a list of ingredients, and a "how to use" section to show that the cosmetic is not misbranded, adulterated, or subject to misuse by the buyer.

All these legalities create a dry topic, but it proves a point. Your makeup can be extremely bad for your health. The industry is largely unregulated in terms of ingredients because the final product is labeled as a cosmetic, rather than a drug or supplement. You could be harming your body extensively by using makeup and other cosmetics.

These products could contain toxic ingredients without your knowledge. Cosmetics are also made with many chemical compounds and synthetics instead of natural ingredients. Anyone who uses cosmetics could be burning their skin, dehydrating it, leaving it open to skin cancers, or poisoning themselves.

There is simply not enough regulation when you consider that a product can enter the market without being checked. For those who do suffer from cosmetic related issues, it can also be extremely difficult to make a complaint. The only law against certain ingredients is that it cannot be adulterated. This means it cannot contain deleterious or poisonous substances, putrid or decomposed substances, or be packaged in an unsanitary condition where it might be contaminated. However, since the FDA does not have to perform checks of all products before they are released, it is difficult to say that each product on the market doesn't have defects. Even all natural ingredients can have defects when not grown in sanitary conditions such as a lab.

Chapter 2: Toxic Ingredients in Your Makeup

Grab one of your products from your makeup bag. Does it have a label? If so, what are the ingredients? Chances are, if you read the ingredients, most of them are chemical names you have never even heard of. What may be worse is that the label may have come off with the wrapping as in the case of eyeliners—if it even had an ingredient label to begin with. You will often see a list of ingredients with the words: "**may contain.**" Does it really contain all of those ingredients? Or just maybe? It is scary to think of what you might be putting on your face everyday. Here are some of the makeup label ingredients that are toxic with long term exposure.

Talc

Next to dioxin, the worst ingredient is Talc. Talc powder often contains asbestos, which has been ruled a highly dangerous toxin. When it is found in houses, a team of professionals have to come in and remove it with special equipment. Yet, women have put it on their faces for decades. Asbestos causes mesothelioma, a cancer that does not appear right away. A woman can be diagnosed with the cancer 30 years after being exposed to it.

PEG

PEG, known as polyethylene glycol, contains dioxin. It is found in personal care products as well as the baby care and sunscreen products that you and your children are using.

Phthalates

According to studies, phthalates are xenoestrogens which are known hormone disruptors. They are in perfumes, hair sprays, skin care lotions, nail polishes and cosmetics. If used enough, they can cause damage to the kidneys, liver or even cause birth defects.

BHA/BHT

BHA/BHT has been found in food as well as makeup products. BHA stands for butylhydroxyanisole and BHT stands for butylhydroxtoluene. In high doses, both of these compounds can impair blood clotting. When large amounts are applied on the skin, they can lead to carcinogenic effects (they can cause cancer).

Dioxin

Do you know what is scarier than named ingredients? The unnamed ones. Dioxin is usually listed under PEGs, which are supposed to be antibacterial ingredients. Yet this is a super-toxic chemical that can cause nervous system disorders, birth deformities, and miscarriages. It is also known to cause cancer. Even the tiniest amount can cause damage to the skin.

Color and Pigment

FD&C color pigments are synthetic colors used in makeup products. The main ingredient to the color and pigment is coal tar. Coal tar is known to contain heavy metal salts, which can cause irritation and skin sensitivity. Certain colors can be absorbed through the skin, which causes oxygen depletion. During animal studies, it was found that these toxic color pigments contained carcinogenic properties, meaning they caused cancer.

DMDM Hydantoin

This is formaldehyde. It is often found in hair conditioners, shampoos, hair gels, cosmetics and skin care products. It is used as a preservative, but tests have found that it can cause a type of dermatitis due to an allergic reaction. It can lead to reddened skin that scales and is difficult to correct.

Diazolidinyl Urea and Imidazolidinyl Urea

Both are formaldehyde concoctions used as preservatives that, again, lead to contact dermatitis due to allergic reactions. In extreme cases, skin grafts to repair the damage have been necessary.

DEA

An ingredient called diethanolamine, or DEA, is a liquid made from fatty acids in coconut oils. It undergoes a chemical reaction used to help thicken shampoo, facial cleansers, and body wash. The chemical process makes this a toxic ingredient that causes skin irritation in addition to liver and kidney cancer. It has also been linked to miscarriages.

When chemistry is applied, even unassuming ingredients, like fatty acids from coconut oils, can have damaging effects to your body, whether it is to your skin or your reproductive system.

Chapter 3: Guidelines for Oils and Skin Types

Choosing the best carrier oils for your skin can be overwhelming. In this book, you will need to use specific carrier oils, according to your skin type, when creating your homemade cosmetics. Here is a list of carrier oils,

specifically for your skin type, along with their properties and benefits.

Jojoba oil- It is the closest to natural skin oils; that is why it's great for all skin types but recommended for those with oily to acne prone skin. It is moisturizing and contains vitamin E. Jojoba oil also balances sebum production and shrinks pores.

Olive oil- Olive oil is good for all skin types but especially dry and mature skin. It contains fatty acids and has anti-inflammatory properties. It's molecules tend to be a little too big for the skin to absorb and can leave an oily feeling.

Sweet almond oil- It is good for all skin types, especially itchy, dry and normal skin. It has a rich source of vitamins and minerals such as vitamin E and D.

Evening primrose- This oil is good for all skin types especially mature, dry and sensitive skin. It contains omega 6 and has antioxidant properties; it is also an anti-inflammatory.

Rosehip seed oil- Rosehip seed oil is a great moisturizer for dry, damaged and dehydrated skin. It is also great for mature skin because of the retin-A that it contains. It also regenerates skin cells. Rosehip seed oil has the potential to lessen the appearance of scars, wrinkles, stretch marks and sun damaged skin.

Avocado oil- This is for all skin types especially mature, dry and sensitive skin and for relieving skin irritations and really dry skin disorders such as eczema and psoriasis. It contains amino and fatty acids and high amounts of vitamins A, B1, B2, D, and E.

Kukui nut oil- It is good for all skin types especially normal, dry and mature skin. Kukui nut oil is packed with vitamins A, C and E. It is specifically used to treat very dry skin.

Wheat germ oil- It is great for mature skin, stretch marks and scar tissue. It's packed with vitamin A and vitamin E as well as unsaturated fatty acids. Wheat germ oil also contains antioxidant properties.

Grapeseed oil- This oil is good for all skin types, especially oily to acne prone skin. It is very lightweight and penetrates the skin very well.

Apricot oil- It is good for all skin types especially normal, dry, aging and sensitive skin. Apricot oil contains high amounts of vitamin A and absorbs quickly into the skin.

Virgin coconut oil- Virgin coconut oil is used for very dry skin and is also great for hair treatments. Always chose unrefined virgin coconut oil; refined oil lacks a lot of nutrients. It locks in moisture and creates a protective hydrating barrier on the skin.

Tamanu oil- This oil is very healing and therapeutic for the skin. It is great for scarred, damaged or dry skin. Tamanu oil is also used to treat skin disorders such as acne, eczema and psoriasis. It accelerates cell regeneration and is anti-fungal.

Normal skin

Jojoba
Sweet Almond
Apricot

Sensitive

Apricot
Grapeseed
Kukui Nut
Avocado

Oily/Acne prone skin

Grapeseed
Jojoba

Combination

Grapeseed
Jojoba
Apricot

Scars/Damaged skin

Kukui Nut
Jojoba
Tamanu
Rosehip Seed

Dry/Mature skin

Jojoba
Kukui Nut
Avocado
Rosehip Seed
Sweet Almond
Tamanu
Olive

Essential Oils

Unlike carrier oils, essential oils are too strong to apply directly to the skin and can cause irritations. They are meant to add natural fragrance to cosmetics but still need to be used according to your skin type. You can always feel free to add a few drops to your DIY products.

Essential Oils for Different Skin Types

Oily to combination skin: orange, lemon, lime, bergamot, geranium, cypress

Acneic skin (to calm and prevent breakouts): tea tree, geranium, vetiver, lavender, patchouli

Dry skin: orange, cedarwood, myrrh, sandalwood, palmarosa, chamomile

Mature (aging skin): tangerine, ylang-ylang, cypress, patchouli, lavender, sandalwood, palmarosa, rose, frankincense

Dark spots: lemon, lavender, orange

Sensitive skin: jasmine, gentle baby

Chapter 4: Homemade Foundation

Creating homemade foundation is not an exact science. It will actually require you to experiment in order to get the right tone/color for your skin. This chapter will require a little patience considering the various aspects that go into making the foundation for your skin type, color, and preferences.

Powder Foundation

The idea behind creating a powder foundation is to design it so that it looks natural, not caked on and does not make your skin appear dry. You must always use a coffee grinder to grind your powders and make them fine enough for application purposes. Since we are working with natural products, the application process can be a little different than what we are normally used to. The powdered foundations tend to get a little messy. Be sure to apply your makeup before getting dressed or cover yourself with a towel.

All Natural Powder with Arrowroot or Cornstarch

You will need arrowroot or cornstarch powder for this recipe. Arrowroot and cornstarch are ingredients that you will run into often with DIY makeup recipes. Arrowroot is a white powder made from a plant. It is added to moisturizers as a thickening agent and to activate the ingredients in order for them to penetrate the skin. Cornstarch (also a white powder) is finely ground corn flour often used as a thickener in cooking. Throughout this chapter, I recommend using arrowroot over cornstarch because more and more people tend to have sensitivities to corn. You'll also need one, some, or all of the ingredients from the following list:

- Ground Cinnamon
- Nutmeg
- Cocoa Powder
- Ground ginger

These ingredients determine the color of the powder foundation that you will choose according to your skin type. You might even need to mix some of them together. If you add too much, you can add in more of your white powder (arrowroot or cornstarch). There are no specific measurements to this recipe; you'll want to slowly add the ingredients to the arrowroot or cornstarch powder in order to get the right consistency and test the color. To get a head start, you can begin by adding:

- 1 teaspoon of cocoa powder
- 1 teaspoon of ground nutmeg
- 2 teaspoons of arrowroot or cornstarch
- ½ teaspoon of ground ginger
- 2 teaspoons of cinnamon

Always grind the powders together in a coffee grinder.

By now you will have experienced all four of the recommended spices as well as the arrowroot or cornstarch powder. From here you will have more of an idea of whether you should add more or less of a specific spice or powder, depending on your skin color.

If you have a store bought foundation, you can try to match it first. Then, work on modifying the color until it is perfect with your skin tone. It's all about mixing and matching until you reach your desired color.

Apply your DIY powder foundation with a kabuki brush for best results!

Chapter 5: Homemade Blush

Powdered Blush Recipes

Whether you are tired of paying for a tiny container of blush in the stores, or you simply want to ensure your health and safety, homemade blush can be the right answer. It is also a simple cosmetic for you to make. You can ensure you are no longer exposing your skin to toxins by using some of the following ingredients:

- Beet powder
- Cornstarch
- Nutmeg
- Ginger

Rosy Cheeks

In a coffee grinder, grind 2 tablespoons of beet powder. Apply a very tiny amount to your cheeks. Apply gradually and go from there to avoid looking like a circus clown. If you would like a smoother application, then disregard the first recipe. Simply mix ½-1 tablespoon of cornstarch to 3 tablespoons of beet powder and grind them together. Although, I prefer the first recipe!

Mauve Blush

- 2 ½ teaspoons of beet powder
- 1 teaspoon of arrowroot or cornstarch
- 1 teaspoon of nutmeg powder

Combine the above ingredients and grind the resulting mixture in a coffee grinder.

Warm Brown Blush

- 1 tablespoon nutmeg
- 1 tablespoon cinnamon
- 1 tablespoon cornstarch

Grind the powders in a coffee grinder.

Golden Brown Blush

- 1 tablespoon of nutmeg
- 1 tablespoon of cinnamon
- ½ tablespoon of cornstarch
- 2 tablespoons of ground ginger

Grind them all together in a coffee grinder

Lilac Blush

- 3 tablespoons cornstarch
- 2 tablespoons beet powder

Grind in coffee grinder

*In most cases, nutmeg tends to darken the blush, while ginger provides a lighter color. Always test the powder on your arm or the back of your hand to see if the color is too dark or too light for your skin tone.

Cream Blush Recipes

A cream blush gives a great, natural, finished look and will last longer than a powder. It is also very pigmented. Simply add 50 drops of carrier oil (see chapter 3) to one of your powdered blushes from the above; "Powdered Blush Recipes" and stir until the mixture becomes creamy.

*Apply this blush in patting motions. Trying to apply it like a regular store blush will make it appear very blotchy, whether in powdered form or especially in cream texture. Your DIY blush may appear blotchy even while properly dabbing it onto your cheeks and can sometimes have grains in it from the powdered spices. The trick is to gently wipe away and remove the grains as you apply it.

Pink Baby Doll Cream blush

Start by adding 4 tablespoons of cornstarch or arrowroot in a bowl and slowly add some beet juice to the powder. Stir until you have a nice, pink, creamy texture. Scoop it up and place it into a tiny lip-gloss container. Allow it to dry for a couple of hours.

Chapter 6: DIY Bronzer

Bronzer is meant to provide a natural suntanned look with some golden shimmer. It's usually applied on areas of your face where the sun would naturally hit, for example: cheeks, nose, chin and sides of the forehead. Here is one fantastic homemade bronzer recipe.

The Ultimate DIY Bronzer Recipe

For a powdered bronzer, you will need:

- 1 teaspoon of cocoa powder
- 1 teaspoon of ground nutmeg
- 1 teaspoon of cornstarch or powdered sugar (powdered sugar will offer a more natural glow or shimmer)
- ½ teaspoon of ground ginger
- 2 teaspoon of cinnamon

Grind the powders together in a coffee grinder.

Although there is no specific, exact mixture for everyone's skin tone, we can agree that bronzer is pretty much a universal color. That's the color I was able to achieve with this combination of spices. It will be, more or less, the same color as your usual bronzer!

Chapter 7: DIY Eyeliner

Eyeliner is meant to enhance the eyes and sometimes even change their shape. Perhaps you are tired of paying for the toxic, costly products you find in your local stores. Finding an eyeliner you can make on your own starts with a few simple ingredients that you probably already have at home. You also need a little container to store your new eyeliner in, as well as a proper eyeliner brush.

Black Gel Liner

All you really need is activated charcoal and a little oil such as avocado, almond, or jojoba. Add the oil one drop at a time until a perfect, creamy, gel texture is reached. The most popular oil for the eye area is castor oil. The oil helps make the eyeliner more like the gel texture that you are used to from the store bought options. Just a few drops into the charcoal and you have a ready-to-use eyeliner. The oil choices are skin friendly and designed to help you remove the makeup easier.

Browning it Up

A lot of the ingredients you already have in your home make great makeup and DIY beauty product solutions, including cocoa powder. If you love to bake and have this item on hand, then you can create your own DIY eyeliner in a brown shade. You want to limit the amount you make to a tablespoon of cocoa powder and a few drops of oil. You can also just wet the brush with oil and apply the powder on that way. It stays long enough for a night out.

A Coconut Option

You can create a different recipe using a few more ingredients. It begins with:

- ½ teaspoon of melted coconut oil

- ½ teaspoon of aloe vera gel
- 2 activated charcoal capsules (for black) or 1 teaspoon of cocoa powder (for brown)

Just mix up the ingredients and store in an airtight container. The coconut oil has health properties while the aloe vera gel makes it easier to remove without irritating the skin around the eyes. Apply the liner onto your eyes and wait a few seconds before applying the second or third coat. Apply as many coats as you need to get your desired shade but don't rub too hard or it will be too translucent.

As you have noticed throughout this eyeliner chapter, there are really only two ingredients that you actually need. In the event that you have nothing else on hand, cocoa powder and oil will make a nice eye liner. You could never go wrong with this option!

Recap on how to apply your DIY gel liner:

Dab the liner onto your eyelid, and add more than one coat as it doesn't quite glide on as smoothly as the eyeliner that you are used to. You need to dab while gliding, and you will need to wait a few seconds before putting on your second or third coat.

If you do not want to use oil, you can substitute with water instead, but I prefer the oil. With water, the color comes out pretty translucent; with the oil, it's very opaque and concentrated just like a real eyeliner.

Chapter 8: DIY Mascara

Mascara is a definite must ladies! You want long and beautiful lashes, but how can you possibly give up mascara that is full of toxins? How can you replace it with a DIY option? Since long, beautiful lashes are a necessity, there are four recipes below that offer you some great ways to not only enhance your lashes but to help them grow longer as well. You can clean out an old mascara tube and brush thoroughly with baby shampoo and apply your homemade mascara inside the tube by creating a tiny funnel (place your mascara in a Ziploc bag and cut the corner of the bag). For a second option, you can simply store your diy mascara in a small container and apply your mascara with a disposable mascara brush.

Seaweed Mascara

This recipe requires:

- 1 tsp of activated charcoal
- 1/8 tsp of ground dried seaweed
- 1/8 tsp of Vitamin E oil
- 1 tbs of shea butter
- 1 tbs of coconut oil
- 1 1/2 tbs of beeswax

Combine all the ingredients into a pan on a hot stove or double boiler. Warm the ingredients until the beeswax melts and the oils mix. It takes 30 to 60 minutes for the mixture to cool and thicken before it can be used. Coconut oil helps keep the mixture from drying out, while Vitamin E provides antioxidants. The charcoal makes the mascara black, while the seaweed is purported to have health benefits and shea butter is very moisturizing.

Warning: According to some research, bladderwrack might be dangerous to use due to the high volume of heavy metals in the water where it grows naturally and is often harvested from. However, this research is not definite. If you know where your seaweed is coming from and you trust that the source has tested it for heavy metals, then you can still use it.

Clay and Aloe Vera Mascara

You need:

- 2 tsp of aloe vera
- 3 capsules of activated charcoal
- 1 tsp of Kaolin clay

You will mix all the ingredients together. Aloe vera is a calming and healing ingredient. The clay will help your mascara to last long and the charcoal is to give it the color. It is definitely better to have that around your eyes than chemicals that could cause sties or redness.

Vegan Mascara

For this recipe, add enough water to 1 tsp of cornstarch until it becomes a type of melted wax texture. Start adding enough castor oil until it turns into a gooey paste (around 10 drops or more). Then add 1 capsule of activated charcoal for the color. The castor oil is going to keep the mascara pliable on your lashes as well as promote hair growth, while the cornstarch helps make it thick enough to glide and stick.

Shea Butter Mascara

Using:

- 1 tsp of coconut oil

- 1 tsp of shea butter
- 1 ½ tsp of beeswax
- 4 tsp of aloe vera
- 1 to 2 capsules of activated charcoal

You will need to heat up and liquefy the coconut oil, beeswax and shea butter in a double boiler. Add the aloe vera and activated charcoal after pouring the liquid in a container once it has cooled down.

Chapter 9: DIY Eye Shadow

How did women beautify their faces before synthetic, chemical factories mass produced makeup? They did so with natural ingredients they found to dye clothing and create paint colors. Plants are the only natural ingredients you need to find all the colors of the rainbow for your eye shadows. You will discover a method to create wonderful eye shadow. It takes a few base ingredients and then a little experimentation to get the exact color you are going for. Go back to your roots, literally, and discover some amazing new colors that are perfect for your skin tone.

The Recipe

Begin with ½ teaspoon of arrowroot or cornstarch powder, ¼ teaspoon of shea butter and 1/8 teaspoon of your powder color of choice. You will need to whisk the shea butter into the powders. You might need to add more shea butter or more powder depending on your results. The finished product will be a heavy, creamy type of powder. If you need to add more spice, keep adding 1/8 teaspoon at a time.

The Colors

The following is a list of potential colors to achieve pinks, yellows, oranges, blacks, greens, browns, blues, purples and so forth. They come in a variety of ingredients that you may already have as well as options that you can find in nature around you.

- Cocoa powder
- Activated charcoal
- Paprika powder
- Nutmeg powder

- Beet powder
- Rose powder
- Geranium powder
- Hibiscus powder
- Bluebell powder (or any flowering plant)
- Ginger powder
- Cinnamon powder
- Cumin powder
- Powdered spirulina
- Curry powder

Combining Ingredients

As you may have noticed, the list of colors uses some spices you probably already have. Obviously some are spicier than others. This means that you want to be careful when applying those as an eye shadow. The idea is to add just enough to get the color you want. The good news is that you can play around a little and experiment until you get the tone you are looking for.

If you feel the color is too bold or too dark, all you need is to add more arrowroot or cornstarch, which will tone it down. Beware that some of these spices can stain your clothes, they can also stain your skin temporarily, if this is the case for your skin, remove with lemon juice!

Chapter 10: DIY Primer

When you use primer before applying foundation, you increase the longevity of your makeup, especially when using DIY products. Your primer can ensure the foundation powder remains on your face throughout the day and makes your foundation appear more vivid. Find out some of the best natural recipes for primers that will help keep your skin looking beautiful. Here is a recipe that does not use already made, synthetic ingredients for primer, which is why the suggestions here ensure you are leaving the toxins behind in favour of all-natural ingredients.

Aloe Vera with Almond Oil

You will need:

- 1/2 tablespoon of water
- 1 tablespoon of fresh aloe vera gel
- 2 drops of almond oil (or substitute jojoba oil for oily to acne prone skin)

Mix and apply the primer evenly on your face. Let it sit for 5-10 minutes before applying makeup. Putting a primer on your face should be done with care. Aloe Vera is an anti-inflammatory, which can help with redness as well as reduce inflammation and pores. You want primers that allow your skin and pores to continue breathing rather than clogging because your skin isn't getting enough oxygen.

Chapter 11: Homemade Cleansers and Moisturizers

Cleansers and moisturizers are an extremely important part of your beauty regime. You want to find a cleanser that will cleanse your face based on the skin type you have and based on the ingredients it contains. When it comes to moisturizers, you have to be careful not to add too much oil to the mixture. You really want a light product to allow your skin and pores to breathe. With these factors in mind, the recipes in this chapter are some of the best choices.

How to Cleanse the Skin:

Gently massage your cleanser onto the skin for about 60 seconds before rinsing with lukewarm water.

Baking Soda Cleanser for Acne Prone Skin

Baking soda works wonders as an at-home acne treatment. It not only exfoliates the skin by opening up clogged pores and scrubbing away dead skin but it's alkaline substance gets rid of any bacteria in the skin that is responsible for causing acne. Simply create a paste like substance by combining baking soda and water in your hand until it is perfect. Massage the paste very gently onto your face before rinsing.

Lemon Juice and Honey for Oily to Combination Skin

Lemon is a natural source of vitamin C; it helps even out and brighten the skin. It also exfoliates and removes acne scars. Honey is antibacterial and works as an anti inflammatory. Honey also helps absorb impurities from the skin. Oatmeal will help to calm the skin and is great for any type of skin irritation.

You will need:

- ½ cup of rolled oats
- ¼ cup of lemon juice

- ½ tablespoon of honey
- ¼ cup of water

Oatmeal and Aloe Vera Juice for Sensitive Skin

Oatmeal and aloe vera are known for treating sunburned or irritated skin, which makes this combination perfect for reducing redness and inflammation caused by sensitivities. Create a pasty substance by adding oatmeal and aloe vera juice together in your hand until it is perfect and solid enough to apply to your face.

Oil Cleansing Method for Dry and Mature Skin (OCM)

The OCM is best suited for dry and mature skin. (See Chapter 3 for some oils best suited for this skin type).

Take some oil of your choice and massage it all over your face. Rinse with warm water to ensure all the oil residue comes off.

The OCM is not for everyone. Do a patch test, for about 2 weeks or more, to see if any break outs occur. If not, continue and you will love your skin, guaranteed!

Refreshing Mint and Yogurt Cleanser for Normal Skin

You will need:

- 2-3 mint leaves (crushed)
- ½ of a small, peeled cucumber (pureed)
- ½ cup of plain yogurt

Simply mix the ingredients together in a bowl. Massage the cleanser into your skin before washing it off.

The mint will leave your skin feeling clean and refreshed. The yogurt is more of a bonding agent for the ingredients and has lactic acid that will brighten the skin naturally. Cucumbers are known to reduce inflammation, particularly dark circles and puffiness.

Sugar and Honey for Dehydrated Skin

Honey is a natural hydrant for the skin. Sugar is great for exfoliating any dead skin on the surface. Honey and sugar together will add a youthful glow to the skin.

You will need to blend sugar, honey and distilled water together until you have a perfect, creamy consistency.

Homemade moisturizers

Applying a daily and nightly moisturizer is a crucial part of your skin care routine. A moisturizer is responsible for locking moisture in the skin as well as keeping or adding elasticity and collagen. It will prevent or eliminate wrinkles; it will nourish and hydrate your skin. It can also reduce or calm sensitive skin or skin inflammations due to acne. Unfortunately, a lot of the skin moisturizers in the stores have tons of parabens and other ingredients that actually do more harm than good. Fortunately, I share with you one great trick to create a skin cleanser specifically made for your skin type.

Here's a very simple DIY moisturizer recipe that you can create for your skin type.

You will need to mix:

- 5 tablespoons of aloe vera gel
- 1 tablespoon of carrier oil according to you skin type (refer to Chapter 3)
- 1 tablespoon of arrowroot or cornstarch powder

Vitalizing Green Tea Serum

A serum is meant to be applied just before your moisturizer and sometimes under a face mask. Serums are lightweight and contain concentrated ingredients. These active ingredients penetrate deeper into the layers of the skin than a regular moisturizer would but are not as moisturizing as a regular face cream. Store bought serums usually carry a hefty price tag, but thankfully you can make the real deal straight from your kitchen cabinets.

Pour boiling water over a green tea bag placed inside a cup. Let it brew for 5 minutes, then allow it to cool. Add ¼ tablespoon of the green tea liquid into your homemade moisturizer from the recipe above.

Chapter 12: DIY Toners

There is an assumption that a toner is not necessary, but in my opinion it is especially important for people with oily skin. It will also remove any remaining dirt left behind that your cleanser didn't remove on its own. Synthetic products can actually do more harm than good, due to the alcohol and glycerin contained within. The recipes in this chapter will not have any ingredients that can irritate your face. The idea is to balance the pH for healthy skin. You will need to bottle the liquid and refrigerate it.

Green Tea and Vinegar Recipe for Oily/Acne Skin

This is a very simple toner that combines acidic and alkaline properties. What this means is that you have an acidic compound like apple cider vinegar that is balanced out with a product that can act as an alkaline base like green tea. You need ¾ cups of green tea, which has been steeped and then ¼ cup of apple cider vinegar. Mix them together. Green tea has anti-inflammatory properties that help with acne, redness, and puffiness. The vinegar helps to lower the pH levels in your skin, if you are prone to oily or acne skin.

Rose Bud Toner for Normal Skin

For this recipe, you need ½ cup of dried rose buds and hot water. You should filter the water. You will need to steep the rose buds like you would tea, except you will steep them for 1 to 2 hours. This is a rose water toner that not only balances the pH of your skin but will also improve dry or irritated skin. It's a soothing mixture that has been used for centuries.

Adding in Geranium Oil for Dehydrated to Dry Skin

The next toner takes the rose water from the above recipe and adds in geranium essential oil. Geranium oil is known to aid hydration. It is a moisturizing element that can repair your dry skin. All you need is a few drops.

Sensitive Skin

You will need 3-4 fresh dried camomile flowers and one cup of boiling water. Add the water to the flowers in a heat resistant container.

Anti-Aging Toner

This is the same as the sensitive skin chamomile toner, only this time you are going to add in a few drops of vitamin E oil. Vitamin E essential oil is known for two things: antioxidants and anti-aging properties. Many makeup products use Vitamin E to help rejuvenate and tighten the skin. Always shake the mixture before applying it to your skin.

Chapter 13: DIY Face Masks

Face and hair mask recipes should be chosen by the type of skin you have. Skin types include combination, dry, mature, normal, oily, and sensitive. You may also have skin issues such as acne, brown spots, dark circles, rosacea, wrinkles, or facial hair that you want to take care of with the proper face mask recipes. All of these face masks should be applied to the face for twenty minutes before rinsing.

All skin types

Turmeric is great for all skin types. It can eliminate acne and provide that rejuvenating boost. Turmeric will brighten the skin and get rid of dark circles, fine lines and wrinkles. It's good for treating skin conditions and even helps remove facial hair. Your face can turn yellow after this mask. There is no need to worry; simply squeeze some lemon juice onto a cotton pad and clean your face. It will come right off!

Mix:

- 2 teaspoons of turmeric powder
- 1 teaspoon of rice or chickpea flour
- 2 teaspoons of plain yogurt
- ½ teaspoons of honey

Combination, Oily, Acne Prone Skin:

Lemon and Sugar Mask

Mix:

- ½ a lemon (lightens acne scarring and evens skin tone)

- ½ a cup of brown sugar (exfoliant)
- 3 tablespoons of honey (moisturizing and antibacterial)

Squeeze the lemon into the brown sugar along with the honey and mix!

Strawberry Chocolate Face Mask

Throw all of these ingredients into a blender:

- ½ cup of water
- 2 tablespoons of cocoa powder (antioxidant, repairs damaged skin, helps with acne)
- 2 tablespoons of Indian healing clay (absorbs oils from the skin and cleans pores)
- 3 medium-sized strawberries (scrubs off dead skin cells, great for acne)
- 1 ½ tablespoons of aloe vera gel (soothes skin)
- A few drops of honey (anti-bacterial, anti-fungal, deeply moisturizing)

It will be a tad runny, but it will start to harden a little on the skin.

Papaya Face Mask

The natural acids in the papaya are mild exfoliants and will brighten up the skin. It contains enzymes that are good for fighting acne.

Mash together:

- 1 ripe papaya
- 4 small strawberries
- 1 teaspoon of lemon juice

Egg White Face Mask

You will need:

- 1 egg white
- 1 teaspoon of lemon juice
- A face brush

Eggs have a lot of protein and nutrients that are great for nurturing the skin. The acid contained in lemons are great for acne scars.

Separate the yolk from the egg white. Stir the egg white and make it really fluffy before adding the lemon juice. Apply the mask with the face brush.

Honey and Cinnamon Face Mask

This recipe is an old Indian creation that mainly uses honey and cinnamon. Honey is known for its antibacterial properties, which helps to disinfect the skin as well as reduce and heal acne spots. Cinnamon is known to help with wrinkles and stimulate hair growth. It helps in numerous ways when digested.

Use 3 tablespoons of honey and 1 tablespoon of cinnamon to create a paste. Layer the mixture over your face before washing it off with warm water.

Sensitive Skin

Egg and Oatmeal Mask for Sensitive Skin

Egg whites can nourish your skin and shrink the pores without leaving your face oily or dehydrated. Oatmeal is not just a high-fibre meal, it is also an ingredient for a number of dry skin issues. Oatmeal also has a hydrating and calming effect on the skin, which is why it is often used in numerous beauty products.

You will need:

- 1 egg white
- 1 teaspoon of oatmeal
- 1 teaspoon of honey

You need to beat the egg white until it turns foamy before adding in the honey and oatmeal. Mix it well and spread it all over your face.

Olive Oil and Honey Face Mask

You will need:

- ½ teaspoon organic raw honey (unprocessed)
- ½ teaspoon extra virgin olive oil

Mix the honey and oil together in a bowl and apply all over your face!

Aloe Vera Face Mask

The best way to do this is to take pure aloe vera from the actual aloe vera plant. Cut the leaf by slicing it in half. Rub the actual leaf onto your entire face. Aloe vera is great for sensitive or sun burnt skin, wrinkles and acne prone skin. Wait 20 minutes and remove.

Rice Milk Sheet Mask

Rice milk is an ancient remedy to soothe and nourish skin. Honey has antioxidants and antimicrobial properties.

Add:

- 1/8 cup of rice milk
- ¼ teaspoon of honey

Add the ingredients in a bowl and microwave for 20 seconds. Take a paper towel and draw a face on it; eyes, a nose and lips. Then, fold it in half and cut out the shapes.

Soak the paper towel in the liquid and apply it to your face!

Mature Skin

Firming and Tightening Wonder Mask

You will need:

- 1/2 a banana
- ½ an avocado
- 1 tablespoon of plain natural yogurt

Mix the ingredients together and leave it in your fridge for a nice, cooling effect. Apply it all over your face.

Coffee Tightening Face Mask

Mix together:

- 1 tablespoon of plain yogurt
- 1 tablespoon of ground coffee (reduces puffiness, tightens skin, reverses free radical damage)

Apply for 10-15 minutes.

Nourishing Milk and Pear Mask

Pear has vitamins and minerals that are great for the skin. It has retinol, keratin, fibers and proteins that are great for wrinkles and mature skin.

Mix:

- 1 tablespoon of mashed pear
- ½ tablespoon of milk

Dry and Dehydrated Skin

In a bowl mix:

- ½ a banana
- 3 tablespoons plain yogurt
- 1 egg white

Avocado and Honey Mask

You will need:

- ½ an avocado
- ¼ cup of honey

Avocado will nourish and help to heal dry skin and the honey will moisturize.

Cool as a Cucumber Mask for Dry Skin

This mask is great for dry skin. All of these ingredients combined will gently refresh and nourish your dermis!

Mash up and mix together:

- 1/2 cucumber
- 1/2 banana
- 1 tablespoon honey
- 4 tablespoons lemon juice

Normal Skin

DIY Rose Petal Mask

The combination of these ingredients will give an instant glow. They are antibacterial and contain both lactic acid and vitamin C.

You will need:

- 1 rose
- 1 tablespoon rose water
- 2 tablespoons honey
- 1 tablespoon of Greek yogurt

Blend the ingredients in a blender.

Apple and Honey Face Mask

For this simple recipe, you will need to blend the following ingredients:

- 1 peeled apple
- 2 tablespoons of honey

Chapter 14: Shampoo/Conditioner & Hair Treatments

Shampoos and conditioners often contain harsh ingredients as discussed in previous chapters. The fact is, all you really need are natural ingredients for beautiful, shiny, clean hair.

Did you know that taking 2-3 tablespoon of baking soda, combined with one cup of warm water is the simplest and most affordable DIY natural shampoo you can make? Baking soda is sodium hydrogen carbonate, which is what provides the cleaning agent. It helps restore the pH levels of the hair and will clean up product buildup.

Cucumber and Lemon Shampoo

You will need to grind half of a peeled lemon (make sure you remove the seeds) and half of a peeled cucumber together. Add more lemon for oily hair and more cucumber for dry hair. Lemon is a great cleansing agent, while cucumber soothes and cools the scalp.

The Honey Solution Shampoo

You could also create a honey and water shampoo. The water is used to make the honey more pliable. You do need to use raw honey. You will need three tablespoons of water to one tablespoon of raw honey. You have to heat the mixture to help the honey dissolve. It will look watery, but this is the correct mixture. Dampen your hair, using your hands, and apply the honey shampoo. Afterwards, rinse it out and use a conditioner.

Honey offers a better pH balance and corrects scalp issues including dandruff. Honey is also known for its anti-fungal and antibacterial properties. The more you use it, the less frizz you will have and the softer your hair will be. You can also go longer without washing your hair again, usually every other day. Natural oil is still produced, but your scalp is healthier and your hair is cleaner.

*Arrowroot and oats are two ingredients that are good for thickening the shampoo as well as helping reduce the pH issues.

Dandruff Buster

After shampooing with your homemade shampoo of choice, fill half of a spray bottle with apple cider vinegar and the rest with cold water. Spray this solution all over the scalp and leave it for fifteen minutes before rinsing. It smells horrible, but it works if you do it at least once a week.

Whipped Cream Coconut Milk Hair Conditioner (for dry hair)

Coconut oil is often added to conditioners claiming they are all natural, when the truth is easy to see by reading the ingredients listed on the back. For the real stuff, follow the recipe below. Apply evenly all over your hair, especially your ends. Just leave it on for a few minutes and rinse thoroughly. This provides moisture to your hair and scalp without leaving an oily feel.

In a blender add:

- 1 banana (reduces frizz)
- A few drops of aloe vera juice (soothes scalp and reduces frizz)
- 1/2 can of coconut milk
- ¼ cup of avocado oil
- A few drops of tea tree essential oil (fights dandruff)(optional)

Yogurt Conditioner for Oily Hair

In a bowl add and mix:

- Half an avocado
- 2 tablespoons of yogurt (all natural)
- 1 tablespoon of honey

This will help reduce excess oil, nourish and moisturize the hair, as well as repair split ends!

Best DIY Hair Detangler

This is the good stuff. If you struggle with tangled hair, your prayers have been answered. I won't say any more, the results speak for themselves!

You will need:

- 1 tablespoon of aloe vera juice (pH balancing, good for dandruff)
- 3 tablespoons of marshmallow root (slippery texture for easy detangling)
- 1 tablespoon of slippery elm powder (improves volume and strengthens hair)
- 3 cups of water
- 10 drops of rosemary oil (stimulates hair growth and is antifungal)
- 1 teaspoon of your favourite carrier oil (for nutrients, vitamins and healthy fats)
- A spray bottle with 1/3 cup of distilled water
- A strainer
- A funnel
- A bowl or measuring cup

Add the marshmallow root, slippery elm and 3 cups of water to a double boiler. Once it's done and very gooey, let it cool for 5 minutes. Pour the gooey mixture into a strainer and drain it into a bowl or measuring cup. Then, place your funnel into the spray bottle and pour in the mixture. Also add the rosemary oil, aloe vera gel and carrier oil into the spray bottle. Place the cover back onto the spray bottle and shake it all up. Store this in the fridge. This hair detangler will last 2-3 weeks. After 3 weeks, throw it away!

Soak it into your hair and scalp and slide your fingers through your hair to detangle before rinsing.

Egg Yolk and Oil Hair Mask

If you desire longer, more luxurious, voluminous hair, then this recipe is for you! Start by using egg yolk, three oils of your choice and honey. The mixture not only helps rehydrate your hair, but it can also help stimulate hair growth according to users. Castor oil, olive oil and argan oil are necessary to help stimulate and regenerate your hair. Argan oil is an ancient ingredient known to add essential moisture back into your hair. Take one egg yolk, 1 teaspoon of honey, olive oil, castor oil, and argan oil. Mix the ingredients until you have a smooth and runny mixture. You should wet your hair until it is damp, before applying the mask. Apply the mask from the roots to the ends of your hair. Leave it on for 30 minutes, then rinse it out with an all-natural shampoo and conditioner.

Honey and Milk Hair Mask

Honey and milk were used by Cleopatra as a bath soak. You can use it to bathe, but it also works as a hair mask. All you need is 2 tablespoons of honey and 1/2 tablespoon of milk. Mix the ingredients and apply it to your hair. Use a plastic bag and towel to cover your hair. Leave it on for 30 minutes. The plastic bag and towel are meant to keep your head warm, this way the treatment will penetrate better into the hair shaft. After 20 minutes, wash your hair with your all-natural shampoo and conditioner. This recipe is particularly helpful for dyed hair.

Mayonnaise Hair Mask Treatment

The mayonnaise hair mask is for anyone who has dry and damaged hair. If you have curly hair, it will definitely bring your curls back to life. This mask hydrates and repairs hair almost instantly because it is a great source of omega 3 fats. Start by wetting your hair with hot water to allow the mayo to easily penetrate into the hair.

Add some mayo in a container and let it sit outside the fridge for about an hour. The warmer it is, the better it will penetrate. Once you are done, apply a shower cap and then a towel over your head for about 20-30 minutes and rinse.

Warning: Can slightly change your hair color if you have dyed hair. Over usage can also cause dry, brittle hair.

Chapter 15: Lip and Body Scrubs

Lips should be soft and kissable. Sometimes the harsh winters, dry months, and generally unhealthy environments that we live and work in, take their toll. Your body can dry out just as easily as your kissable lips. Having safe and natural DIY scrubs that will rejuvenate your skin is essential. Inside this chapter, you will find recipes using all natural ingredients that you may have lying around the house.

Lime Margarita Mousse Lip and Body Scrub

This recipe can be used for your entire body or just your lips. It is up to you, but the main thing is to remove all that dead skin, rejuvenate it to a moisturized shine and feel great about yourself.

Ingredients:

- 2 teaspoons of coconut oil
- 10 drops kuikui nut oil
- 4 drops lime essential oil
- ½ teaspoon lime or lemon juice
- ½ teaspoon lime zest (optional)
- 2 tablespoons of sugar

Mix the ingredients together. The sugar is what provides the grainy scrubbing power behind the lip and body scrub. Each of the oil ingredients have been chosen for their antibacterial, moisturizing and rejuvenation qualities.

Honey Lip Scrub

Honey is known for its antibacterial properties as discussed in other chapters. It can also add moisture to your skin including your lips. Using one teaspoon of honey and one tablespoon of granulated sugar, combine the ingredients into a paste. Rub the paste on your lips for five minutes before rinsing. Then, use a lip balm to add more moisture. The honey will heal the chapped lips and peel away the dead skin with the sugar granules.

Whipped Shea Butter Body Scrub

Mix together 1 tablespoon of raw shea butter, 10 drops of carrier oil, 1 tablespoon of arrowroot or cornstarch, and 1 tablespoon of sugar. The carrier oils will provide rejuvenating essential vitamins. Cornstarch or arrowroot is important for the consistency of the recipe. The sugar is, of course, going to offer the grainy feel that is required to scrub the dry skin from your body. Shea butter is the most essential ingredient in this recipe because it is going to fix the dry skin issue more than any other additive.

Holiday Gift to Yourself: Peppermint Body Scrub

Want to make a gift around the Christmas holiday? There is a peppermint candy body scrub recipe that is perfect. Take 1 tablespoon of sugar and 1 tablespoon of olive oil with 3 or 4 drops of peppermint oil. Mix all the ingredients together. It will be ready to give as a gift to yourself or a loved one. The peppermint oil is a relaxation additive with a fragrance that makes the scrub smell great. The olive oil is a moisturizer to help reduce the dry skin that is common during winter.

Vanilla Sugar Cookie Body Scrub

I love the smell of fresh baked cookies right out of the oven. If you do too, then here is a fantastic vanilla sugar cookie scrub recipe just for you!

You will need to mix:

- ½ a cup of melted coconut oil
- 2 cups of sugar

- A few drops of vanilla

Add it to a pretty jar and you are done!

Pink Lemonade Body Scrub

Add:

- 2 cups of white sugar
- 2/3 cup of any carrier oil
- 2 teaspoons of lemon juice
- A bit of red beet juice

Stir the first three ingredients together. Add a tad of red beet juice. Start with less and continue adding until it turns into a pretty pink lemonade color!

These recipes are just the tip of the iceberg when it comes to lip and body scrubs. Almost any essential oil can be used with sugar to create a rejuvenating, moisturizing body scrub.

Chapter 16: Homemade Hairspray

In terms of toxic qualities, hairspray has been an issue for decades. Some strides have been made to take out the most flammable chemicals, but it is still not a friend to the environment or your hair. The homemade hairspray recipes found here can provide you with the staying power you need without harming your precious locks. You will need to have a spray bottle on hand that mists liquid out, lightly.

Natural Sugar Hairspray

Add 3 teaspoons of sugar to half a cup of boiling water. The more sugar you add, the stronger the hold. Heat the water and sugar in the pot until the sugar dissolves. Allow the water to cool, then place the hairspray into a spray bottle using a funnel. Let it cool in the fridge for about 20 minutes.

Lemon Lavender Lightening Hairspray

You will need 2 lemons for this recipe. Lemon, is great for lightening hair. If you have darker hair and do not wish to have it lightened, substitute the lemons with oranges. You will also need 2 cups of distilled water, 3 teaspoons of sugar and a few drops of lavender essential oil. You can always substitute a different essential oil, or simply leave it out. Remove the peels of the lemons and cut them in pieces. Then, boil the lemons in the water over medium heat until the liquid is reduced by half. Drain with a strainer into a bowl. Allow the citrus juice to cool. Add the essential oil to the mix before funnelling it into a spray bottle.

How to Use Your Homemade Hairspray: Never apply a whole lot like you would with a regular hairspray; you need to spray in layers and let it dry in between sprays. 2-3 coats usually does the trick! It can last about 2 weeks. If you want your hairspray to last longer than 2 weeks then you will need to add in some alcohol.

Chapter 17: DIY Lipstick and Lip Gloss

Whether you are a lipstick fanatic or all about lip gloss, there are recipes for you to choose from to ensure you are making your own from trusted ingredients.

To add color to your lip gloss or lipstick, all you need are natural powders, spices or Mica powders that are safe for your skin. For example, cinnamon can offer a nice shade of reddish brown. You can add cocoa powder for a deeper shade of brown or beet powder for bright red lips.

For added color, you will need some ground, natural colored powders in your recipe. You can add more or less of it and you might even need to mix them.

You could also check out Chapter 5 for some of the powdered blush recipes that you might like to use as a lip gloss.

Lip Gloss (no Vaseline or beeswax)

This recipe does not include Vaseline or beeswax. It ensures a light and airy feel without the greasy sensation of Vaseline or heavy beeswax.

Start with:

- 1 tablespoon of cocoa butter
- ½ teaspoon olive oil
- 1 tablespoon of honey

You will need to put these ingredients into a double boiler until they become a liquid. Pour the mixture into a small lip gloss container and add a colored powder (optional). Let it harden in the fridge for about an hour. This lip gloss must always be kept in the fridge in order for it to stay solid.

Natural Lipstick with Beeswax

Start off with:

- ½ tablespoon coconut oil
- 1 tablespoon shea butter
- ½ tablespoon beeswax
- 1 tablespoon of powder of your choice (optional)

Melt these ingredients together in a double boiler. Pour the mixture into a container once it has cooled off a little. If you decide to add color, decide which powder you want to use. Get your desired color and mix it in.

Organic Mango Butter Lip Gloss

You will need:

- ½ a tablespoon of coconut oil
- ⅓ tablespoon mango butter
- ¼ tablespoon shea butter
- ½ tablespoon beeswax
- 1 tablespoon of your favourite powder (optional)

Melt the coconut oil, mango, beeswax and shea butter in a double boiler. Add your powder (optional) and put it in jar or empty lip gloss container. Cool it off in the fridge.

Adding Essential Oils

If you want fragrance, you can add essential oils like peppermint, vanilla, rose, lavender and so forth. You always want to add in 1/8 of a teaspoon when you add in essential oils.

Conclusion

Hopefully you have enjoyed these DIY tips. You also gained plenty of knowledge with regards to skin and hair care. It is easy to understand why you might be tired of purchasing chemical laden, synthetic makeup supplies. It is bad for your health and not easy on your wallet.

Now you have solutions that can ensure that your health is a priority. Many of the ingredients are found at home. You don't have to make a big shopping list or hunt for special ingredients because your kitchen most probably has them.

For the ingredients that you may not already have, it is a simple matter. It is reasonable to assume that you might not have cocoa butter, beeswax, shea butter, or some of the more specialized options just lying around. These ingredients are only a health store away. All you need is one organic shop or you can buy online.

Hopefully you will share what you have learned with others and start practising some of these recipes to see which ones work best for you. You have plenty of different options to try.

Since these are homemade recipes, it will take a little playing around, some fun, and definitely some trials. The good news is that at the end of it all, you will have natural DIY makeup and toxin free homemade cosmetics that are certainly not tested on animals, are safe to use and that you can trust.

Enjoy the process, explore, and feel free to share your thoughts. Spread your knowledge with others as you become an expert in creating your very own products.

For a FREE copy of my book;

Face Mask Recipes *60 Homemade Face Mask Recipes For Beautiful, Radiant Skin*

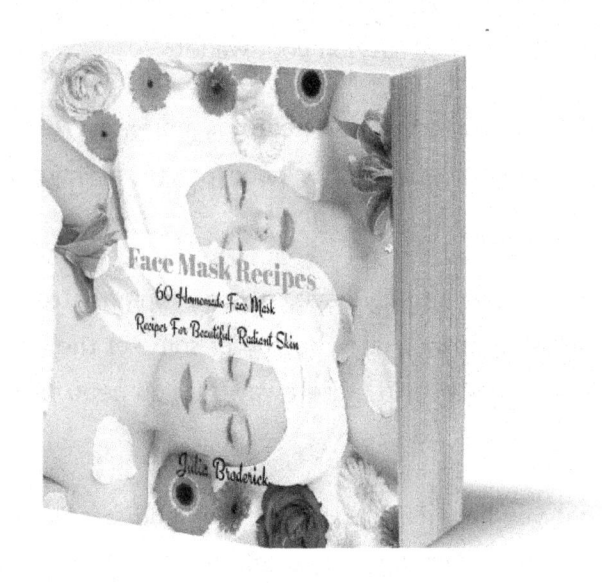

Type the link below into your internet browser:

http://eepurl.com/bWMRZb

Julia Broderick Social Media;

Website/blog:

http://www.beautifulhealthymom.com/

Youtube Channel:

https://www.youtube.com/user/beautifulhealthymom1

Facebook Page;

https://www.facebook.com/BeautifulHealthyMom/

Twitter:

https://twitter.com/Beautyhealthmom

For more books;

http://www.beautifulhealthymom.com/our-products/

Made in the USA
Columbia, SC
03 January 2018